I0116866

30-Day
Wellness Journey:
Mindfulness, Gratitude, Growth

Chichi Nwankwo Ezeike MD/MPH
Certified Integrative Health Coach

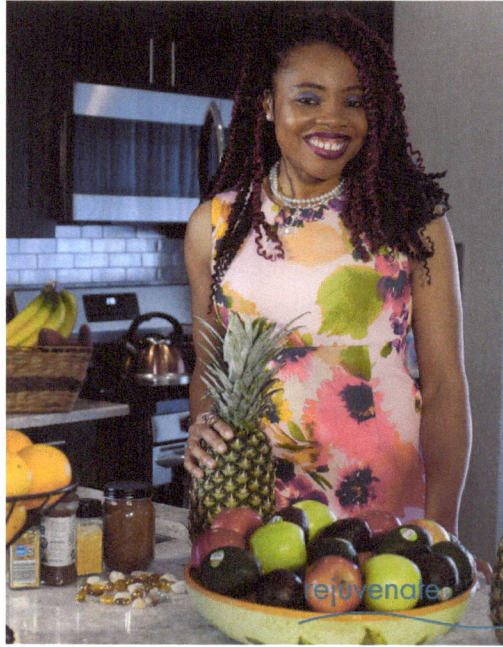

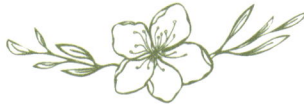

Or do you not know that your body is a temple of the Holy Spirit within you, whom you have from God? You are not your own, for you were bought with a price. So, glorify God in your body.
1 Corinthians 6:19, 20 ESV

30-Day
Wellness Journey:
Mindfulness, Gratitude, Growth
Written by Chichi Nwankwo Ezeike MD/MPH

© Copyright Chichi Nwankwo Ezeike MD/MPH
Published by Pa-Pro-Vi Publishing
www.paprovipublishing.com

Photos taken by Chichi Nwankwo Ezeike MD/MPH

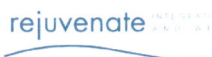

rejuvenate

All Rights Reserved. No part of this book may be reproduced, scanned, or transmitted in any form or by any means, digital, audio or printed, without the expressed written consent of the author.

ISBN: 978-1-959667-67-4
Printed in the United States of America
To reach author, go to www.rejuvenateinhealth.com

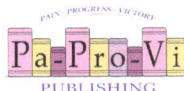

PAIN · PROGRESS · VICTORY
Pa-Pro-Vi
PUBLISHING

DEDICATION

Proverbs 3:8 "This will bring health to your body and nourishment to your bones."

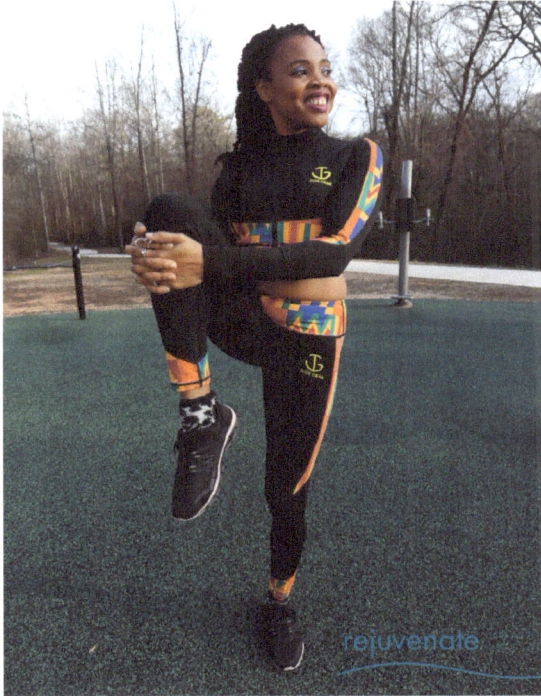

I want to dedicate this 30-Day Wellness Journey to everyone battling to find holistic ways to get healthy. I pray that as you embark on this journey of Health and Wellness, this journal will be an encouragement to you. I pray that you will be strengthened as you meditate on the word of God. As psalm 103: 3b states that "...He heals all your diseases" may you start to receive your healing in Jesus' name.

THANK YOU

I want to thank my Savior and Lord, Jesus Christ for the inspiration to write this journal. I also want to thank my husband, Brian, our 4 children, my siblings, my in-laws, and my friends who continue to encourage me on my health journey.

INTRODUCTION

As a physician and certified health coach, I have come to deeply understand the profound truth behind the saying, "Health is Wealth." However, like many, I did not fully grasp its significance until I was personally confronted with a hypertension diagnosis. That moment forced me to reflect on the countless patients I had treated—those who suffered from strokes, chronic kidney disease, and other debilitating complications, all stemming from uncontrolled hypertension. I recalled individuals who started with a single prescription, only to find themselves on a cascade of medications, managing side effects rather than addressing the root cause.

That day, I had an epiphany. I realized that conventional medicine alone was not enough—I needed a more comprehensive, proactive approach to combat this silent but deadly disease. My pursuit of a solution led me to the Health Coaching Institute, where I discovered the power of holistic health. Through my training, I realized I was not alone in this quest; there is a growing movement of individuals seeking sustainable, integrative solutions for their well-being.

Armed with both my medical expertise and health coaching principles, I founded Rejuvenate Integrative Health and Wellness—a practice dedicated to empowering individuals to take control of their health through a holistic, sustainable lifestyle. My approach goes beyond symptom management; I educate and guide my clients in embracing wellness as a lifelong journey rather than a temporary fix.

I invite you to embark on this transformative journey with me—one where you define your own path, free from guilt or shame over setbacks. Every step you take matters, and every small victory is a milestone toward greater health. This book is your guide, equipping you with the tools to cultivate mindfulness, practice gratitude, and achieve growth—physically, mentally, emotionally, and spiritually.

Your health is your greatest asset. Let's reclaim it together.

Day 1

Behold, I will bring to it health and healing, and I will heal them
and reveal to them abundance of prosperity and security.
Jeremiah 33:6 ESV

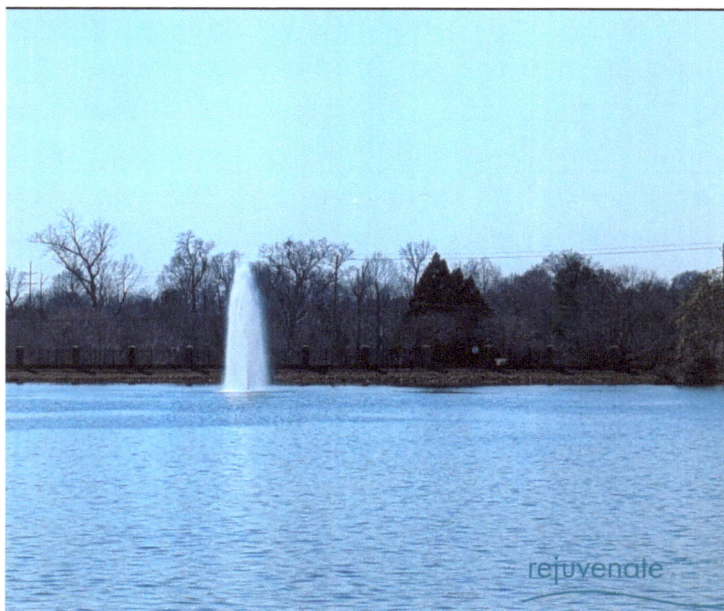

Today's Intentions:

1. Begin each task with a focused attention.

2. Incorporate mindfulness breaks throughout the day.

3. Show gratitude for three things, big or small.

Reflections:

- Starting the day with a clear intentions help you to stay focus and productive.
- Mindfulness breaks allow you to reset and recharge, enhancing your overall well-being.
- Gratitude practice reminds you of the abundance in your life, fostering a positive mindset.

Journal your thoughts

Day 2

You shall serve the Lord your God, and he will bless your bread
and your water, and I will take sickness away from among you.
Exodus 23:25 ESV

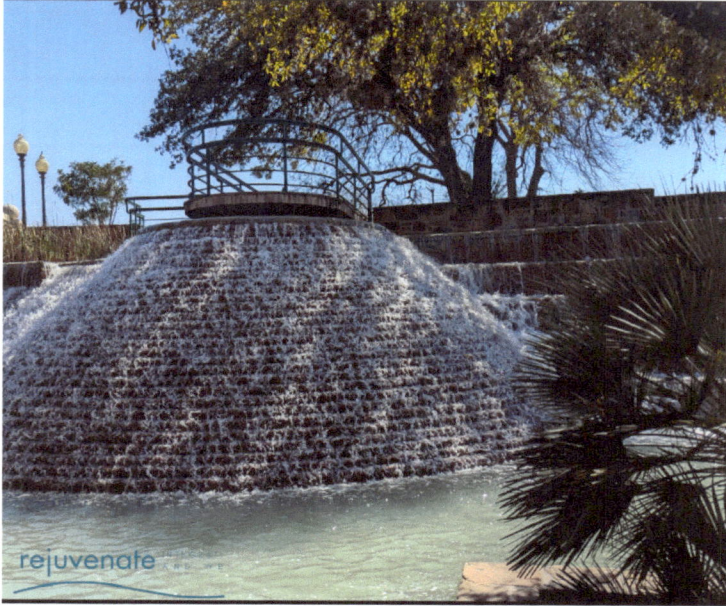

Today's Intentions:

1. Practice deep breathing exercises to reduce stress.

2. Engage in physical activity for at least 30 minutes.

3. Offer support and encouragement to someone in need.

Reflections:

- Deep breathing exercises have proven to be effective in calming your mind and reducing stress levels.

- Physical activity boost your energy and lift your mood.

- Offering support to a friend in need strengthens your bond and brings a sense of fulfillment.

Journal your thoughts

Day 3

A joyful heart is good medicine, but a crushed spirit dries up the bones. Proverbs 17:22 ESV

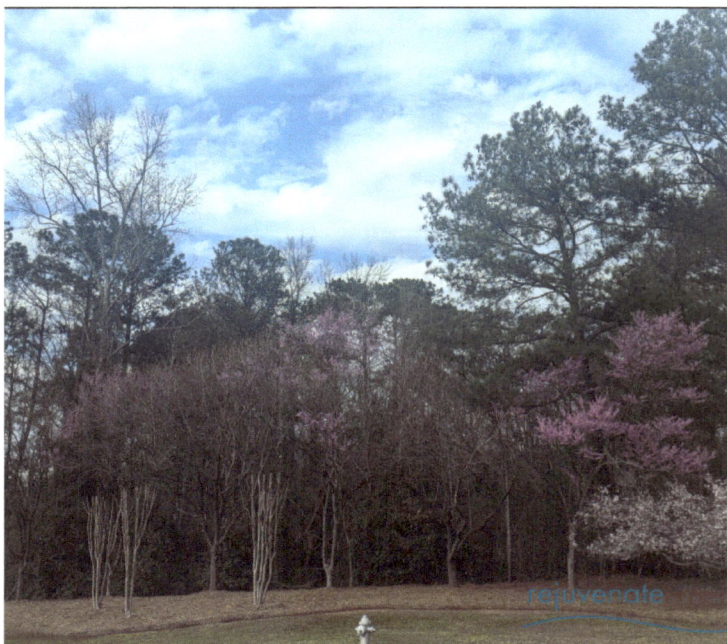

Today's Intentions:

1. Prioritize self-care by getting enough rest and nourishment.

2. Practice positive affirmations to cultivate self-confidence.

3. Engage in a creative activity for personal enjoyment.

Reflections:

- Prioritizing self-care allows you to feel rejuvenated and ready to tackle the day's challenges.
- Positive affirmations boost your self-confidence and helps shift your mindset towards success.
- Engaging in a creative activity sparks joy and enhances your overall well-being.

Journal your thoughts

Day 4

Beloved, I pray that all may go well with you and that you may be in good health, as it goes well with your soul. 3 John 1:2 ESV

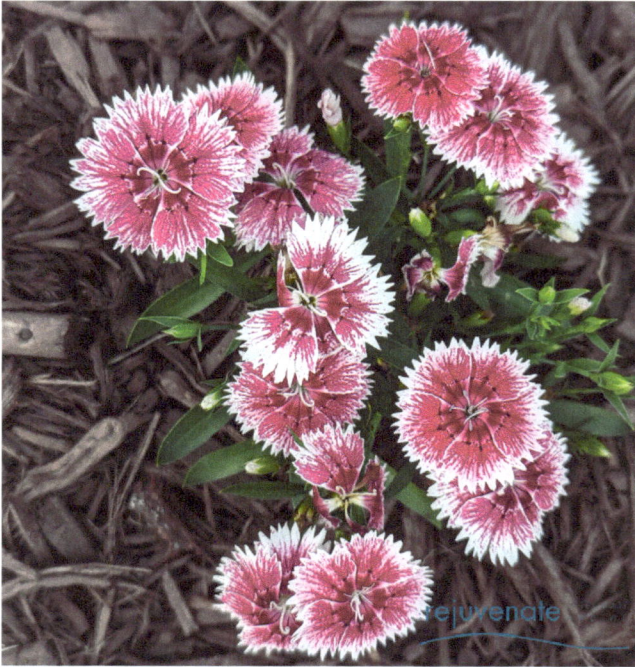

Today's Intentions:

1. Practice active listening in all conversations.
2. Set realistic goals for the day and celebrate small victories.
3. Reflect on moments of joy and gratitude before bed.

Reflections:
- Practicing active listening fosters deeper connections and understanding in your interactions.
- Setting realistic goals helps you to stay focus and motivated throughout the day.
- Reflecting on moments of joy and gratitude before bed fills you with a sense of contentment and peace.

Journal your thoughts

_____

_____

_____

_____

_____

_____

_____

_____

_____

_____

_____

_____

_____

_____

_____

_____

Day 5

But he answered, "It is written, man shall not live by bread alone, but by every word that comes from the mouth of God".
Matthew 4:4 ESV

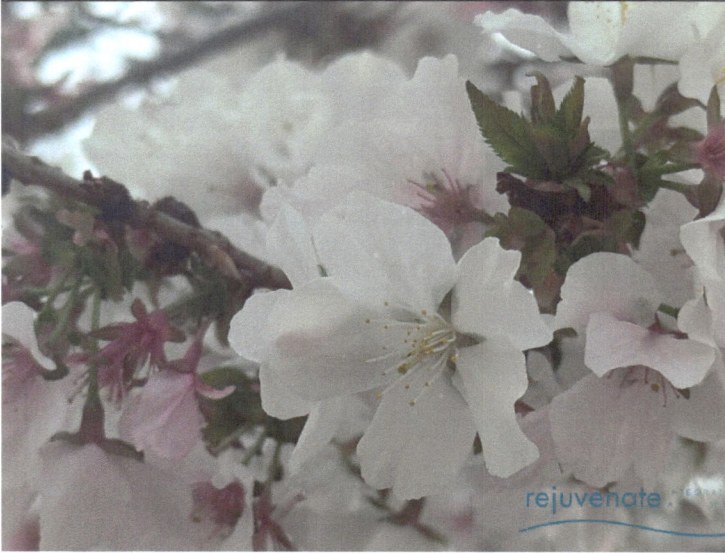

Today's Intentions:

1. Practice forgiveness towards yourself and others.

2. Engage in a random act of kindness.

3. Reflect on areas of personal growth and development.

Reflections:

- Practicing forgiveness allows you to release negative emotions and cultivate inner peace.

- Engaging in a random act of kindness brings joy to both you and others.

- Reflecting on areas of personal growth and development reminds you of the progress you've made and inspires you to continue striving for excellence.

Journal your thoughts

_____

_____

_____

_____

_____

_____

_____

_____

_____

_____

_____

_____

_____

_____

_____

_____

_____

_____

Day 6

Heal me, O Lord, and I shall be healed; save me, and I shall be saved, for you are my praise. Jeremiah 17:14 ESV

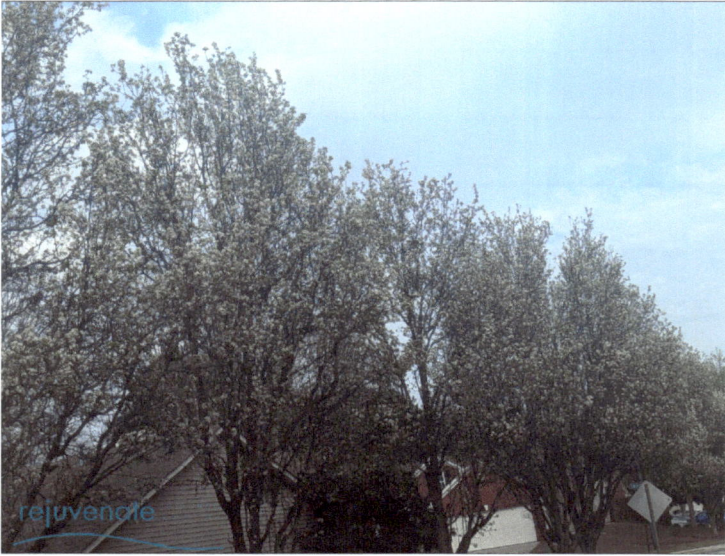

Today's Intentions:

1. Practice mindfulness during daily activities.

2. Engage in a gratitude meditation before bed.

3. Reflect on lessons learned from challenges faced today.

Reflections:

- Practicing mindfulness helps you stay present and fully engage in each moment.

- The gratitude meditation before bed fills you with a deep sense of appreciation for the abundance in your life.

- Reflecting on lessons learned from challenges provides valuable insights and opportunities for growth.

Journal your thoughts

_____

_____

_____

_____

_____

_____

_____

_____

_____

_____

_____

_____

_____

_____

_____

_____

_____

Day 7

Anxiety in a man's heart weighs him down, but a good word
makes him glad.
Proverbs 12:25 ESV

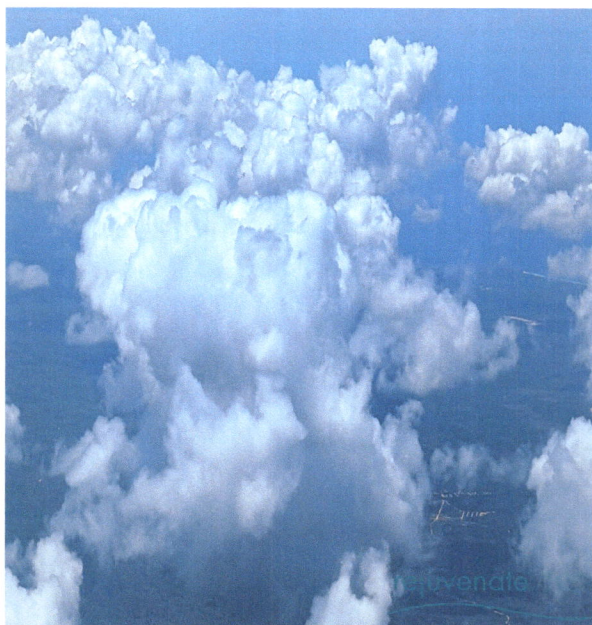

Today's Intentions:

1. Practice deep relaxation techniques before starting the day.

2. Set boundaries to protect your time and energy.

3. Reflect on moments of joy and fulfillment throughout the day.

Reflections:

- Starting the day with deep relaxation techniques set a positive tone and allows you to approach tasks with clarity and focus.
- Setting boundaries helps you to maintain balance and avoid being overwhelmed.
- Reflecting on moments of joy and fulfillment reminds you to savor life's simple pleasures and stay connected to what truly matters.

Journal your thoughts

Day 8

For they are life to those who find them, and healing to all their flesh.
Proverbs 4:22 ESV

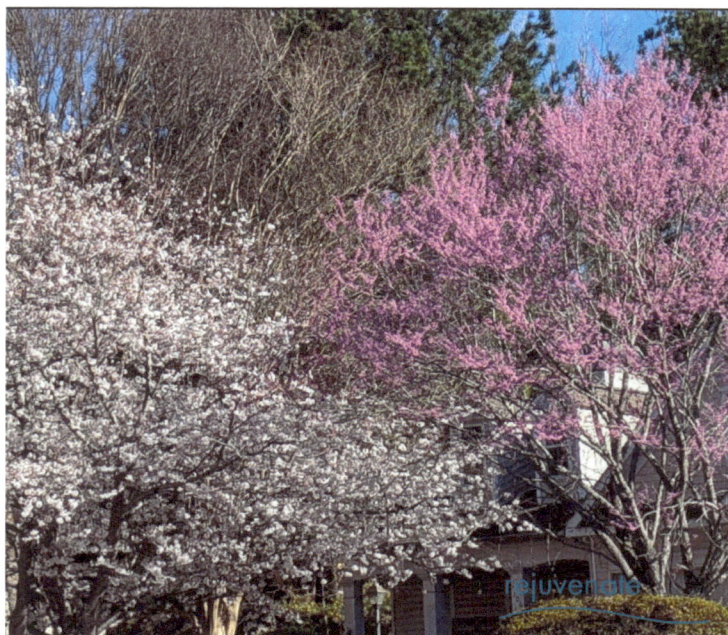

Today's Intentions:

1. Engage in a self-care activity that nourishes your mind, body, or soul.
2. Practice positive self-talk and affirmations.
3. Reach out to a loved one to express gratitude and appreciation.

Reflections:

- Engaging in a self-care activity provides much-needed rejuvenation and relaxation.
- Positive self-talk and affirmations boost your confidence and self-esteem.
- Reaching out to a loved one to express gratitude deepens your connection and fosters a sense of mutual appreciation.

Journal your thoughts

Day 9

So, whether you eat or drink, or whatever you do, do all to the glory of God.
1 Corinthians 10:31 ESV

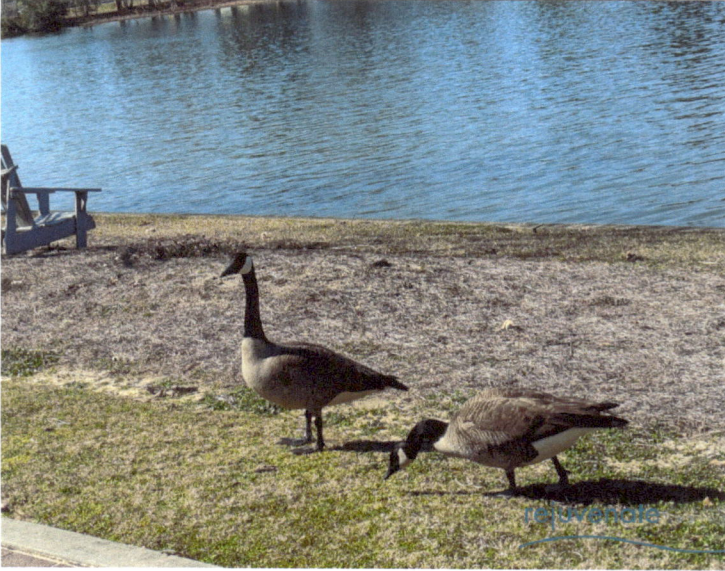

Today's Intentions:
1. Practice mindful eating by savoring each bite and listening to your body's hunger cues.
2. Take breaks throughout the day to rest and recharge.
3. Reflect on moments of resilience and strength.

Reflections:

- Practicing mindful eating enhances your appreciation for nourishing foods and helps you cultivate a healthier relationship with eating.

- Taking breaks to rest and recharge prevents burnout and allows you to sustain energy levels throughout the day.

- Reflecting on moments of resilience and strength reminds you of your inner power and capacity to overcome challenges.

Journal your thoughts

_____

_____

_____

_____

_____

_____

_____

_____

_____

_____

_____

_____

_____

_____

_____

_____

_____

Day 10

If you have found honey, eat only enough for you, lest you have your fill of it and vomit it.
Proverbs 25:27 ESV

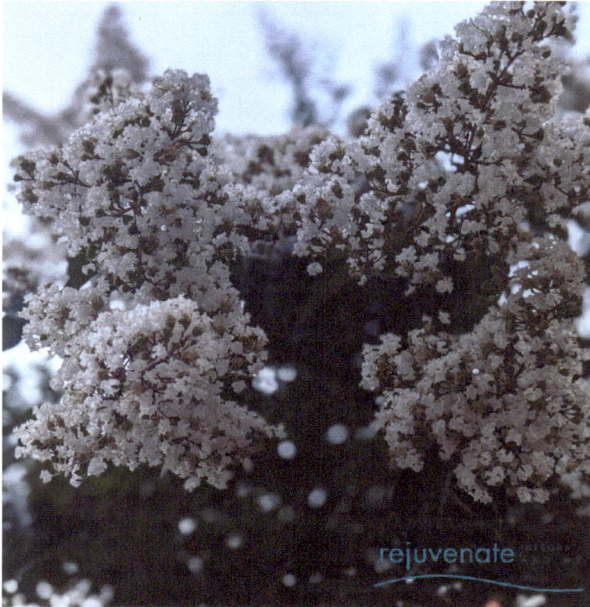

Today's Intentions:
1. Engage in a gratitude journaling exercise.
2. Practice deep breathing exercises during moments of stress or anxiety.
3. Reflect on areas of personal growth and celebrate progress made.

Reflections:
- Gratitude journaling deepens your appreciation for the blessings in your life and fosters a sense of abundance.

- Deep breathing exercises proves effective in calming your mind and reducing stress levels.

- Reflecting on areas of personal growth reminds you of how far you've come and inspires you to continue striving for excellence.

Journal your thoughts

Day 11

"And God said, "Behold, I have given you every plant yielding seed that is on the face of all the earth, and every tree with seed in its fruit. You shall have them for food." Genesis 1:29 ESV

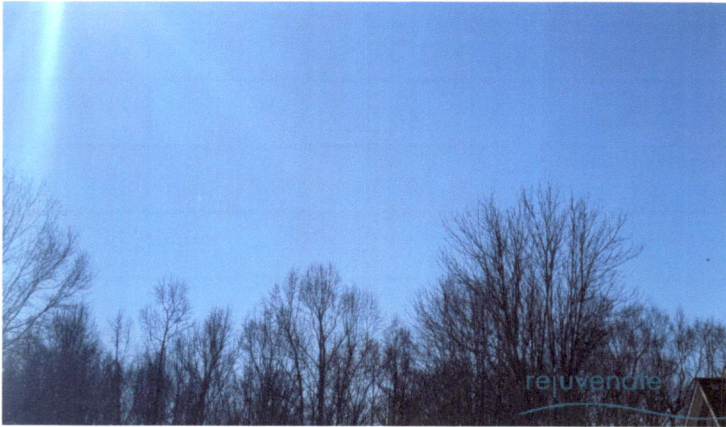

Today's Intentions:

1. Practice active listening in all conversations, focusing on understanding rather than responding.
2. Engage in a physical activity that brings joy and vitality.
3. Reflect on moments of kindness received and extended throughout the day.

Reflections:

- Practicing active listening deepens your connections with others and fostered empathy and understanding.

- Engaging in joyful physical activity invigorates your body and lifts your spirits.

- Reflecting on moments of kindness reminds you of the beauty of human connection and the ripple effect of compassion.

Journal your thoughts

Day 12

But Daniel resolved that he would not defile himself with the king's food, or with the wine that he drank. Therefore, he asked the chief of the eunuchs to allow him not to defile himself.
Daniel 1:8 ESV

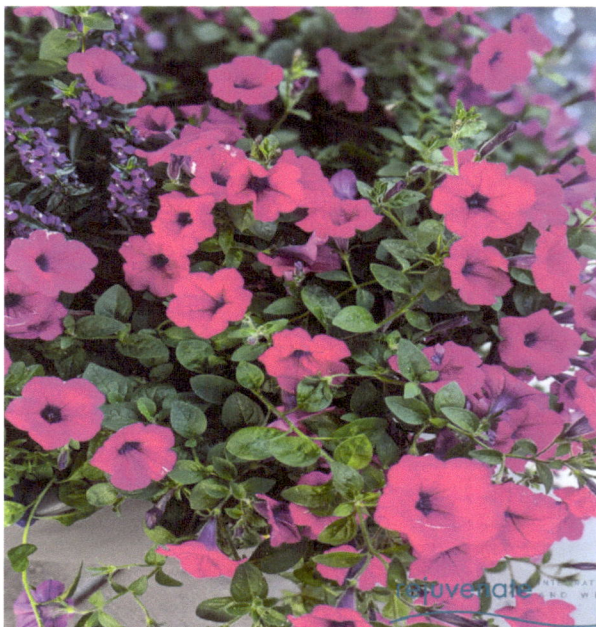

Today's Intentions:
1. Set aside time for quiet reflection and meditation.
2. Identify areas of self-improvement and create actionable steps towards growth.
3. Express gratitude for the lessons learned from challenges faced.

Reflections:
- Quiet reflection and meditation provides clarity and inner peace, it allows you to reconnect with your inner wisdom.

- Identifying areas of self-improvement empowers you to take proactive steps towards personal growth and development

.
- Expressing gratitude for the lessons learned from challenges transforms setbacks into opportunities for learning and resilience.

Journal your thoughts

_____

_____

_____

_____

_____

_____

_____

_____

_____

_____

_____

_____

_____

_____

_____

_____

_____

_____

Day 13

If you will diligently listen to the voice of the Lord your God, and do that which is right in his eyes, and give ear to his commandments and keep all his statutes, I will put none of the diseases on you that I put on the Egyptians, for I am the Lord, your healer. Exodus 15:26 ESV

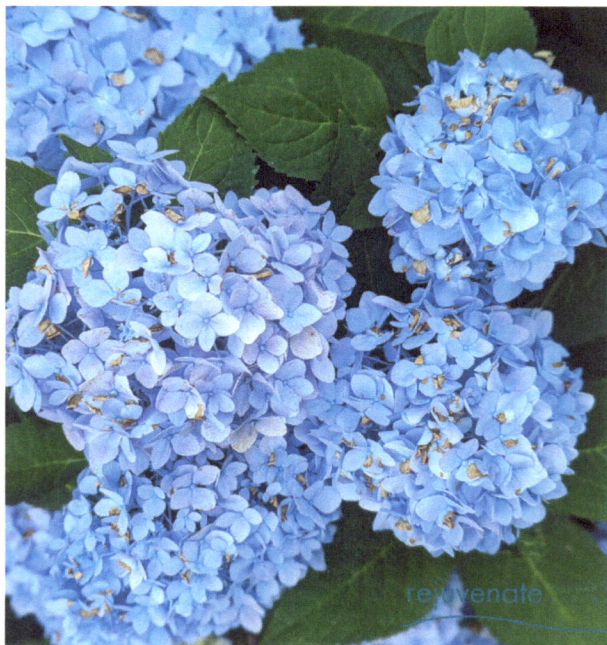

Today's Intentions:

1. Practice visualization techniques to manifest goals and dreams.
2. Engage in acts of self-care that nurture the mind, body, and spirit.
3. Reflect on moments of joy and fulfillment experienced throughout the day.

Reflections:

- Visualization techniques fuels your motivation and inspires action towards manifesting your goals and dreams.

- Acts of self-care replenishes your energy and enhances your overall well-being.

- Reflecting on moments of joy and fulfillment fills you with gratitude and reminds you to appreciate life's simple pleasures.

Journal your thoughts

Day 14

It will be healing to your flesh and refreshment to your bones.
Proverbs 3:8 ESV

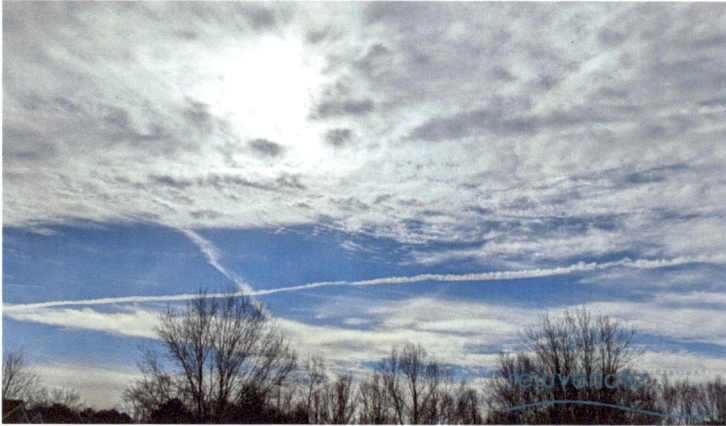

Today's Intentions:

1. Practice compassion towards yourself and others.

2. Set boundaries to protect your emotional and mental well-being.

3. Reflect on moments of growth and progress.

Reflections:

•Practicing compassion fosters a sense of connection and empathy, both towards yourself and others.

•Setting boundaries empowers you to prioritize your well-being and honors your needs.

•Reflecting on moments of growth and progress reminds you of your resilience and capacity for positive change.

Journal your thoughts

Day 15

He gives power to the faint, and to him who has no might he
increases strength.
Isaiah 40:29 ESV

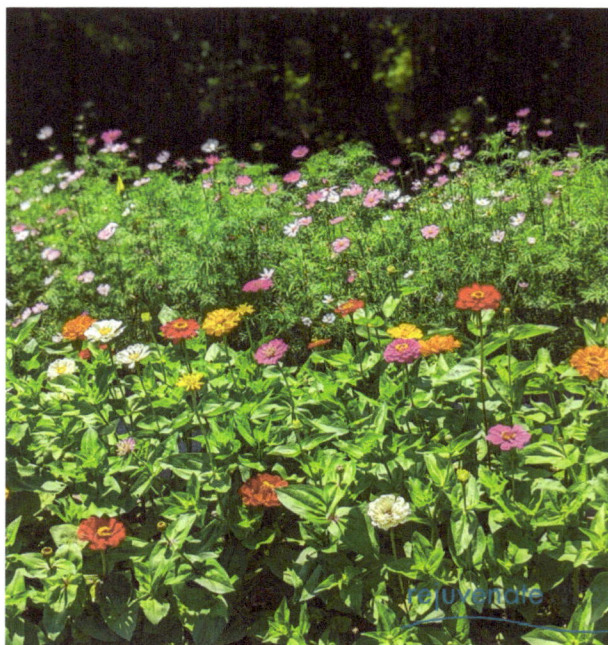

Today's Intentions:
1. Practice mindful communication by speaking with intention
and listening with empathy.
2. Engage in a gratitude practice by acknowledging the
abundance in your life.
3. Reflect on moments of resilience and strength demonstrated
in overcoming challenges.

Reflections:
- Mindful communication enhances the quality of your
  interactions and deepens connections with others.

- Practicing gratitude reminds you of the richness and
  blessings present in your life.

- Reflecting on moments of resilience reaffirms your inner
  strength and resilience in the face of adversity.

Journal your thoughts

Day 16

I appeal to you therefore, brothers, by the mercies of God, to present your bodies as a living sacrifice, holy and acceptable to God, which is your spiritual worship. Romans 12:1 ESV

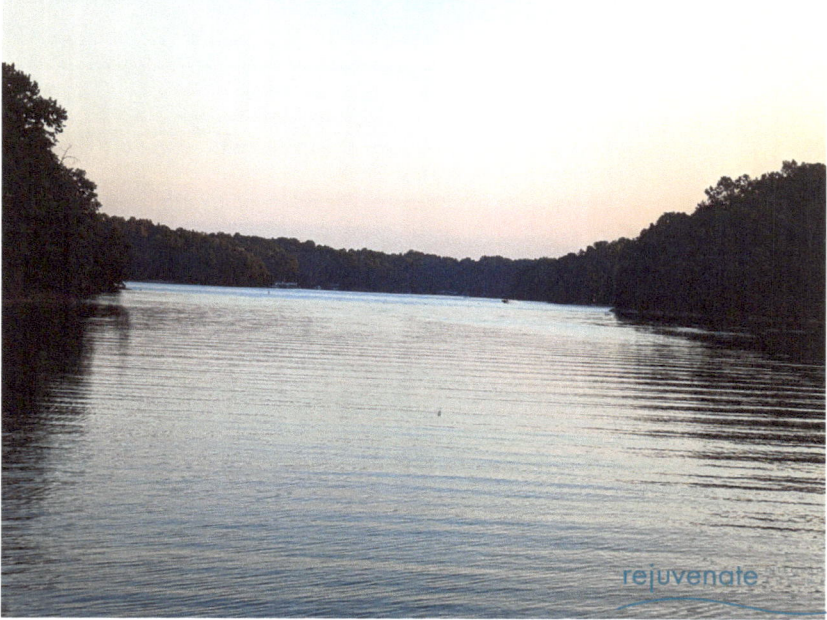

Today's Intentions:
1. Prioritize rest and relaxation to rejuvenate mind and body.
2. Engage in a self-care ritual that promotes inner peace and tranquility.
3. Reflect on moments of kindness received and extended throughout the day.

Reflections:
- Prioritizing rest and relaxation allows you to recharge and approach the day with renewed energy and clarity.

- Engaging in a self-care ritual provides a sense of calm and centeredness amidst life's busyness.

- Reflecting on moments of kindness highlights the beauty of human connection and the impact of small acts of compassion.

Journal your thoughts

Day 17

But for you who fear my name, the sun of righteousness shall rise with healing in its wings. You shall go out leaping like calves from the stall. Malachi 4:2 ESV

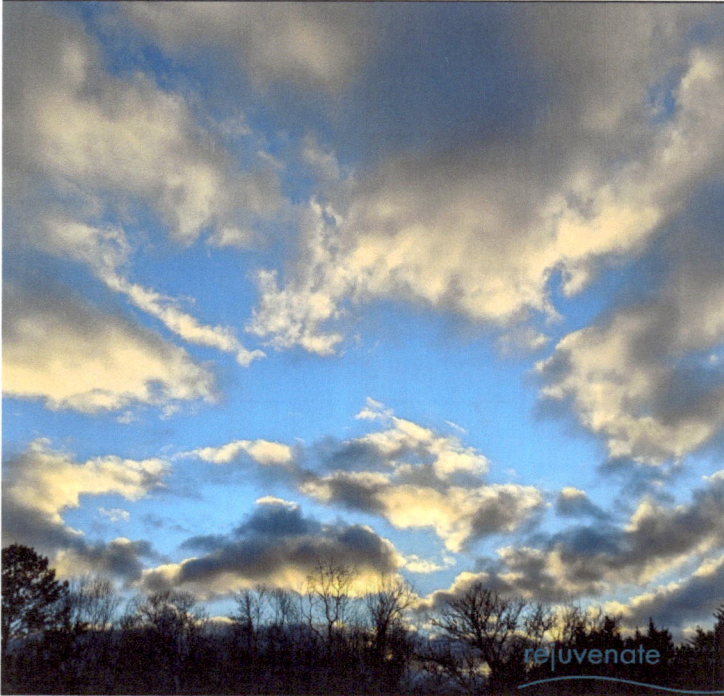

Today's Intentions:
1. Practice gratitude by acknowledging the beauty in everyday moments.
2. Engage in a mindfulness exercise to ground yourself in the present moment.
3. Reflect on areas of personal growth and celebrate progress made.

Reflections:
- Practicing gratitude heightens your awareness of the blessings surrounding you and fills your heart with appreciation.

- Engaging in a mindfulness exercise anchors you in the present moment, fostering a sense of peace and clarity.

- Reflecting on areas of personal growth reminds you of your resilience and capacity for positive change.

Journal your thoughts

Day 18

But they who wait for the Lord shall renew their strength; they shall mount up with wings like eagles; they shall run and not be weary; they shall walk and not faint. Isaiah 40:31 ESV

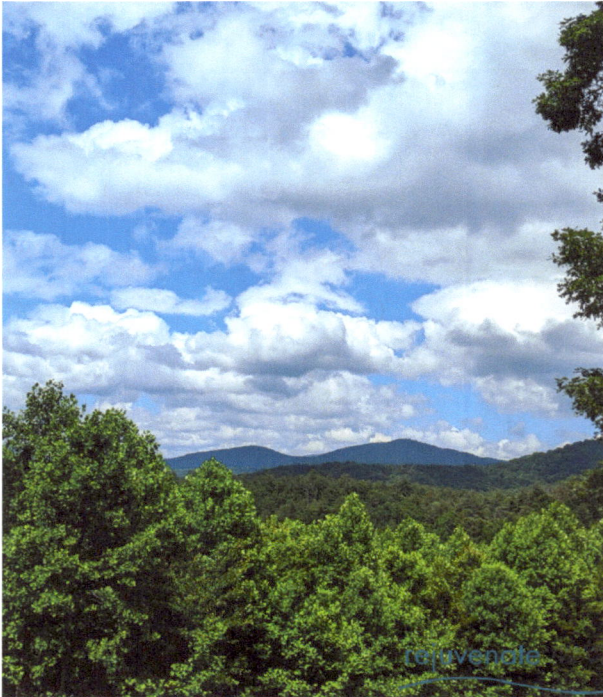

Today's Intentions:
1. Practice self-compassion by treating yourself with kindness and understanding.
2. Engage in a physical activity that energizes and uplifts you.
3. Reflect on moments of joy and fulfillment experienced throughout the day.

Reflections:
- Practicing self-compassion allows you to embrace your imperfections with love and acceptance, fostering inner peace and self-confidence.

- Engaging in physical activity invigorates your body and mind, boosting your mood and energy levels.

- Reflecting on moments of joy and fulfillment fills you with gratitude and reminds you to cherish life's simple pleasures.

Journal your thoughts

Day 19

Is anyone among you sick? Let him call for the elders of the church, and let them pray over him, anointing him with oil in the name of the Lord. And the prayer of faith will save the one who is sick, and the Lord will raise him up. And if he has committed sins, he will be forgiven. James 5:14,15 ESV

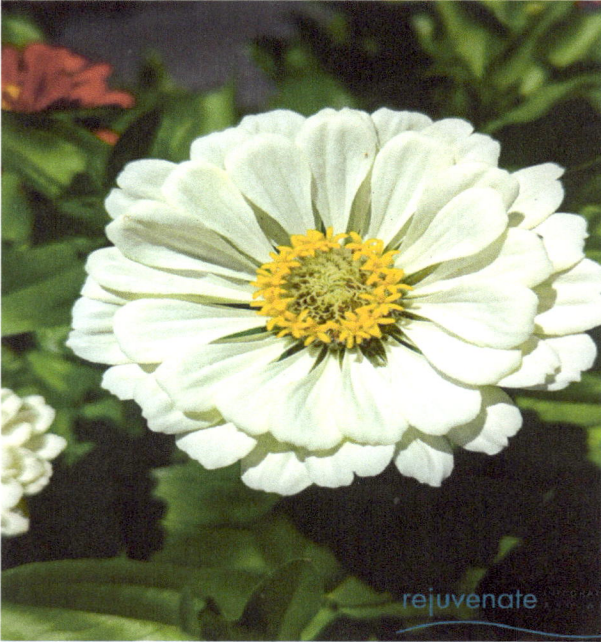

Today's Intentions:
1. Set aside time for creative expression and exploration.
2. Practice deep breathing exercises to promote relaxation and stress relief.
3. Reflect on moments of growth and learning from challenges faced.

Reflections:
- Engaging in creative expression sparks your imagination and provides a sense of freedom and joy.

- Practicing deep breathing exercises calms your mind and body, allowing you to release tension and find inner peace.

- Reflecting on moments of growth and learning reminds you of your resilience and ability to overcome obstacles with grace and strength.

Journal your thoughts

Day 20

He heals the brokenhearted and binds up their wounds. Psalm 147:3 ESV

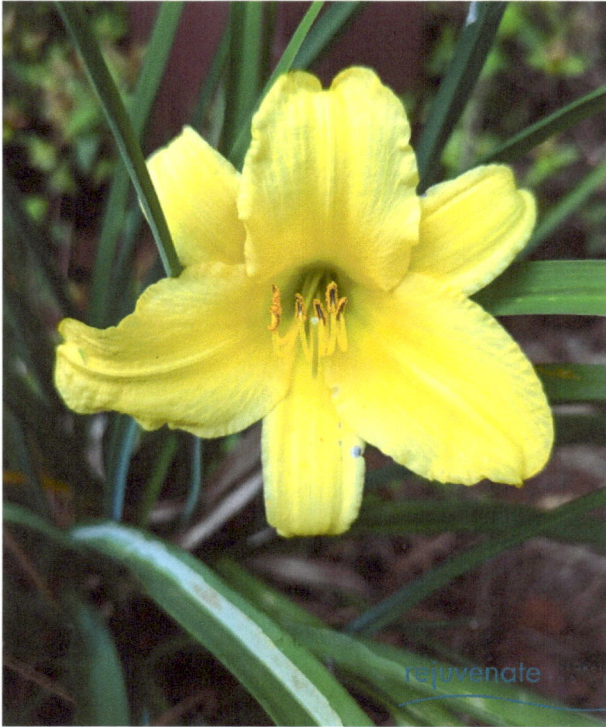

Today's Intentions:

1. Cultivate a positive mindset by focusing on solutions rather than dwelling on problems.
2. Engage in acts of kindness towards yourself and others.
3. Reflect on moments of gratitude and appreciation throughout the day.

Reflections:

- Cultivating a positive mindset empowers you to approach challenges with optimism and resilience, leading to creative solutions and growth.

- Acts of kindness, whether towards yourself or others, creates a ripple effect of positivity and connection.

- Reflecting on moments of gratitude and appreciation fills you with warmth and reminds you of the abundance present in each day.

Journal your thoughts

Day 21

For I will restore health to you, and your wounds I will heal, declares the Lord, because they have called you an outcast: 'It is Zion, for whom no one cares!' Jeremiah 30:17 ESV

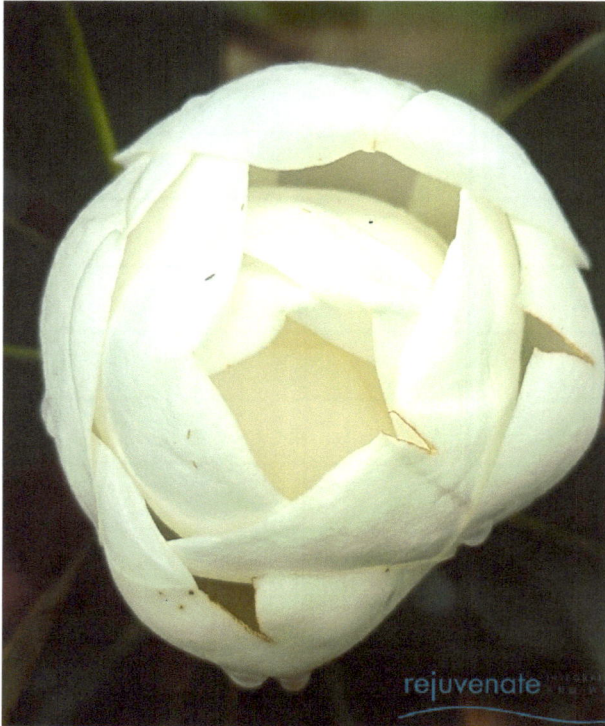

rejuvenate

Today's Intentions:
1. Practice mindfulness during daily activities, bringing awareness to each moment.
2. Set realistic goals for the day and celebrate progress made.
3. Reflect on moments of self-love and acceptance.

Reflections:
- Practicing mindfulness enhances your presence and allows you to fully engage in the richness of life's experiences.

- Setting realistic goals provides clarity and direction, leading to a sense of accomplishment and fulfillment.

- Reflecting on moments of self-love and acceptance deepens your connection with yourself and fosters inner peace and contentment.

Journal your thoughts

_____

_____

_____

_____

_____

_____

_____

_____

_____

_____

_____

_____

_____

_____

_____

_____

Day 22

But when he heard it, he said, "Those who are well have no need of a physician, but those who are sick." Matthew 9:12 ESV

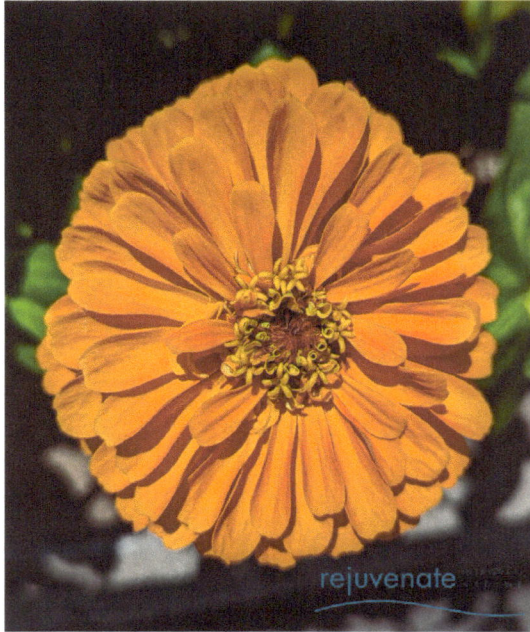

Today's Intentions:

1. Engage in a gratitude meditation to cultivate appreciation for the present moment.
2. Practice self-reflection to gain insight into personal values and aspirations.
3. Reflect on moments of growth and resilience in navigating life's challenges.

Reflections:

- The gratitude meditation deepens your sense of appreciation for the beauty and abundance present in each moment, fostering a profound sense of joy and contentment.

- Self-reflection allows you to gain clarity on your values and aspirations, guiding your actions towards a life aligned with your true purpose.

- Reflecting on moments of growth and resilience reminds you of your inner strength and capacity to overcome adversity with grace and resilience.

Journal your thoughts

Day 23

Test your servants for ten days; let us be given vegetables to eat and water to drink. Daniel 1:12 ESV

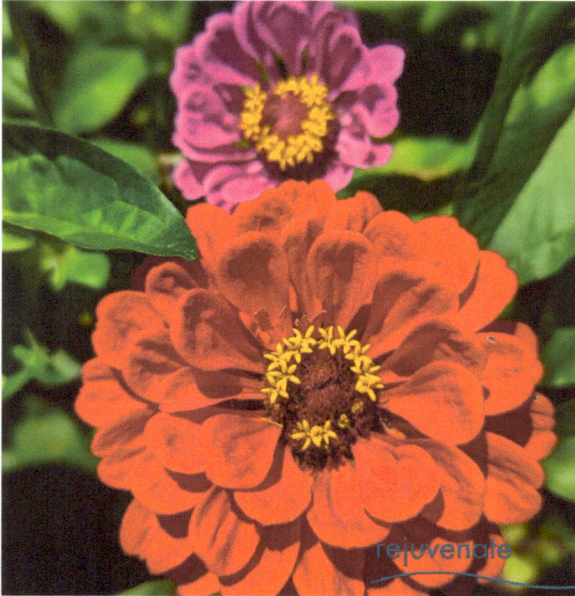

Today's Intentions:
1. Practice forgiveness towards yourself and others, releasing any lingering resentment or judgment.
2. Engage in a mindful walk, connecting with nature and grounding yourself in the present moment.
3. Reflect on moments of kindness received and extended throughout the day.

Reflections:
- Practicing forgiveness liberates your heart from the weight of past grievances, allowing you to experience greater freedom and inner peace.

- The mindful walk immerses you in the beauty of nature, rejuvenating your spirit and fostering a sense of interconnectedness with the world around you.

- Reflecting on moments of kindness illuminates the inherent goodness in humanity and fills you with gratitude for the love and compassion shared between individuals.

Journal your thoughts

_____

_____

_____

_____

_____

_____

_____

_____

_____

_____

_____

_____

_____

_____

_____

_____

_____

_____

Day 24

Now when the sun was setting, all those who had any who were sick with various diseases brought them to him, and he laid his hands on every one of them and healed them. Luke 4:40 ESV

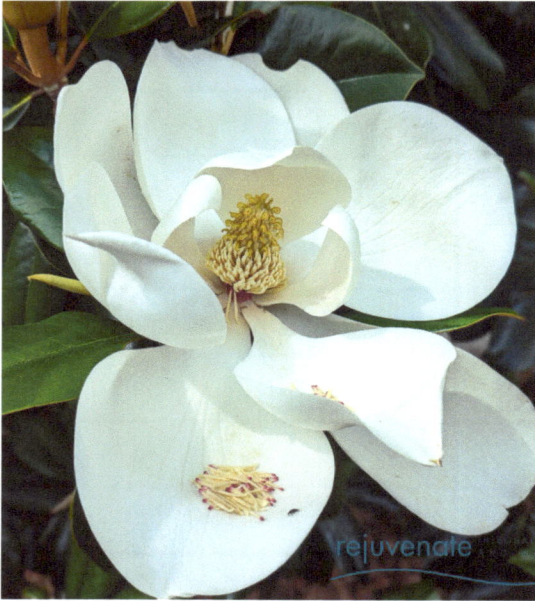

Today's Intentions:

1. Start the day with positive affirmations to set the tone for a productive and fulfilling day.
2. Practice deep breathing exercises to promote relaxation and mental clarity.
3. Reflect on moments of growth and progress, acknowledging the steps taken towards personal goals.

Reflections:

- Beginning the day with positive affirmations fills you with confidence and optimism, laying the foundation for a day filled with possibility and opportunity.

- Deep breathing exercises provide moments of calm amidst the busyness of the day, allowing you to navigate challenges with clarity and composure.

- Reflecting on moments of growth and progress reaffirms your commitment to personal development and inspires you to continue moving forward with determination and resilience.

Journal your thoughts

Day 25

Gracious words are like a honeycomb, sweetness to the soul and health to the body. Proverbs 16:24 ESV

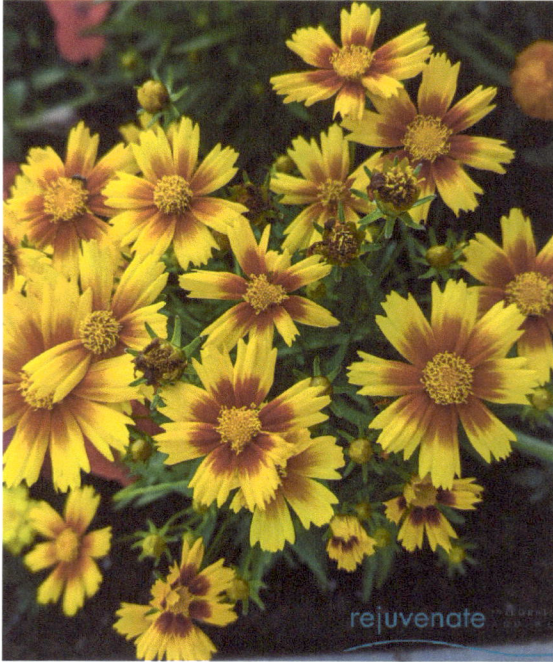

rejuvenate

Today's Intentions:
1. Practice gratitude by expressing appreciation for the people, experiences, and blessings in your life.
2. Engage in a self-care activity that nourishes the mind, body, and spirit.
3. Reflect on moments of joy and fulfillment, savoring the beauty of life's simple pleasures.

Reflections:
- Practicing gratitude fills your heart with warmth and appreciation, reminding you of the abundance of blessings present in your life.

- Engaging in a self-care activity provides a much-needed opportunity for rest and rejuvenation, replenishing your energy and vitality.

- Reflecting on moments of joy and fulfillment brings a smile to your face and reminds you to cherish the beauty of each moment.

Journal your thoughts

Day 26

But he was pierced for our transgressions; he was crushed for our iniquities; upon him was the chastisement that brought us peace, and with his wounds we are healed. Isaiah 53:5 ESV

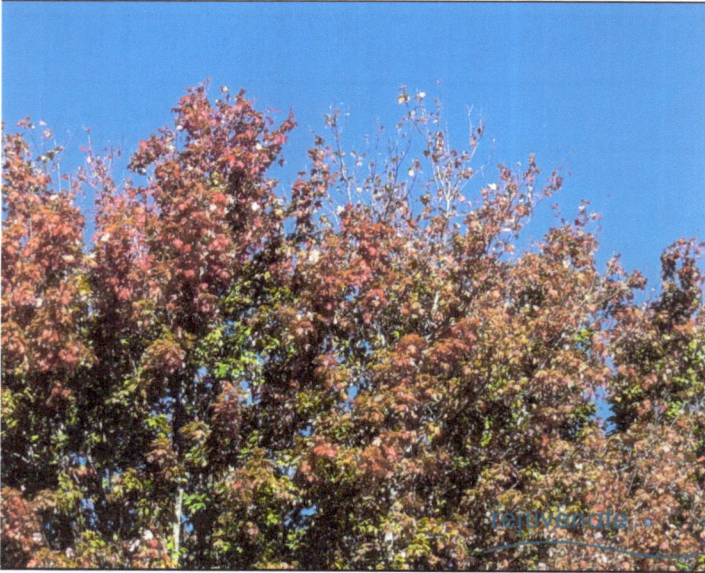

Today's Intentions:
1. Practice mindfulness in all activities, bringing awareness to the present moment.
2. Set aside time for reflection and journaling to gain insight and clarity.
3. Reflect on moments of resilience and strength, acknowledging your inner power to overcome challenges.

Reflections:
- Practicing mindfulness allows you to fully immerse yourself in the richness of each moment, cultivating a sense of peace and contentment.

- Journaling provides a space for self-expression and introspection, helping you gain clarity and insight into your thoughts and emotions.

- Reflecting on moments of resilience and strength reminds you of your inner resilience and capacity to navigate life's challenges with grace and courage.

Journal your thoughts

Day 27

Their fruit will be for food, and their leaves for healing.
Ezekiel 47:12d ESV

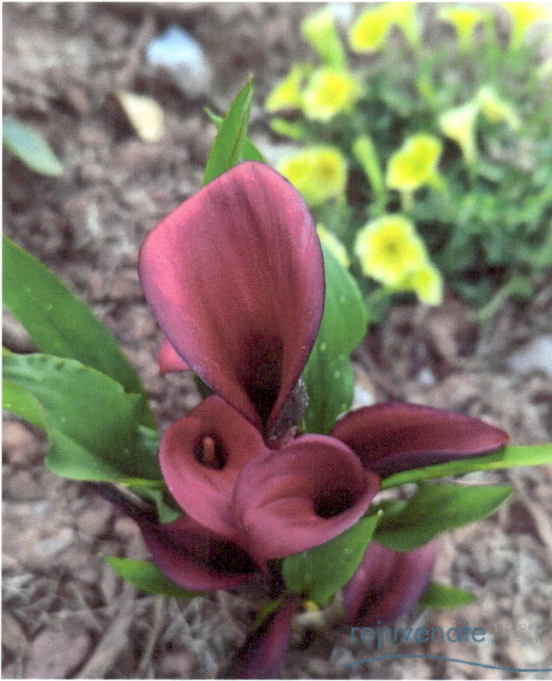

Today's Intentions:
1. Practice self-compassion by treating yourself with kindness and understanding.
2. Engage in a physical activity that brings joy and vitality.
3. Reflect on moments of growth and learning from challenges faced.

Reflections:
- Practicing self-compassion allows you to embrace your imperfections with love and acceptance, fostering a sense of inner peace and self-confidence.

- Engaging in physical activity invigorates your body and mind, boosting your mood and energy levels.

- Reflecting on moments of growth and learning reminds you of the valuable lessons gained from overcoming obstacles, empowering you to continue moving forward with resilience and determination.

Journal your thoughts

_____

_____

_____

_____

_____

_____

_____

_____

_____

_____

_____

_____

_____

_____

_____

_____

_____

Day 28

Jesus turned, and seeing her he said, "Take heart, daughter; your faith has made you well." And instantly the woman was made well.
Matthew 9:22 ESV

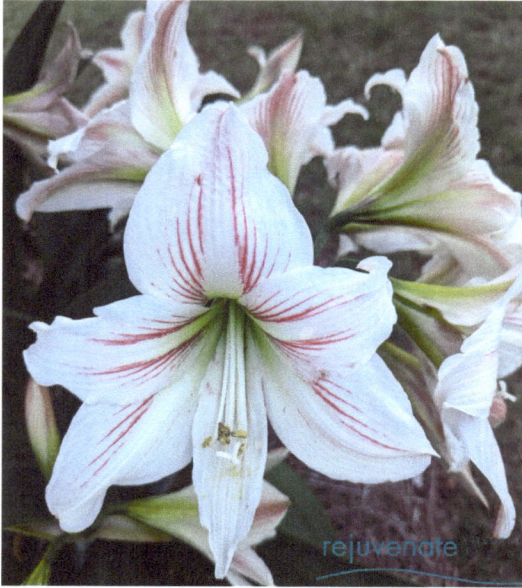

Today's Intentions:

1. Cultivate a mindset of abundance by focusing on opportunities rather than limitations.
2. Engage in acts of kindness towards yourself and others, spreading positivity and compassion.
3. Reflect on moments of gratitude and appreciation for the journey so far.

Reflections:

- Cultivating a mindset of abundance opens your eyes to the myriad possibilities and opportunities surrounding you, filling you with optimism and excitement for the future.

- Acts of kindness, whether small or grand, creates ripples of positivity that enriched both your life and the lives of those around you.

- Reflecting on moments of gratitude and appreciation fills you with a deep sense of fulfillment and reminds you of the beauty and richness of the journey you're on.

Journal your thoughts

_____

_____

_____

_____

_____

_____

_____

_____

_____

_____

_____

_____

_____

_____

_____

_____

Day 29

If my people who are called by my name will humble themselves, and pray and seek my face and turn from their wicked ways, then I will hear from heaven and will forgive their sin and heal their land. 2 Chronicles 7:14 ESV

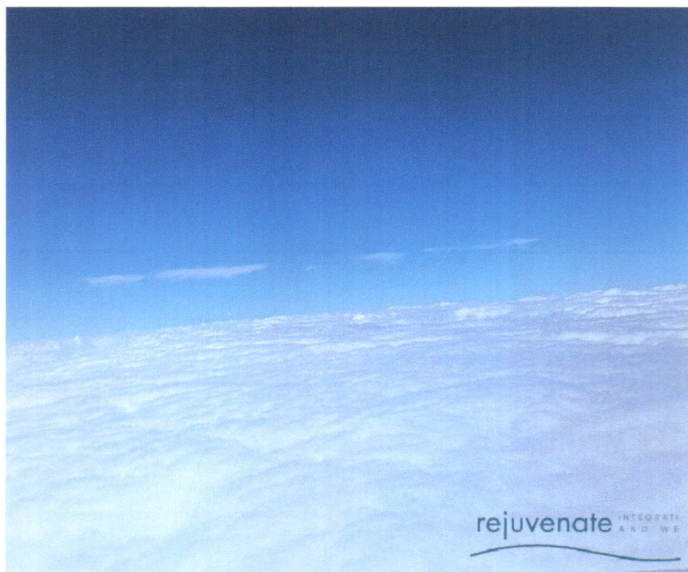

rejuvenate INTEGRATE AND WE

Today's Intentions:
1. Practice mindfulness in daily activities, savoring each moment with awareness and presence.
2. Set aside time for creative expression, tapping into your inner creativity and imagination.
3. Reflect on moments of growth and resilience, recognizing the progress made on your journey.

Reflections:
- Practicing mindfulness infuses each moment with a sense of wonder and appreciation, allowing you to experience life more fully and deeply.

- Engaging in creative expression sparks your imagination and brings forth a sense of joy and fulfillment, reminding you of the importance of nurturing your creativity.

- Reflecting on moments of growth and resilience fills you with pride and gratitude, reaffirming your belief in your ability to overcome obstacles and thrive in the face of challenges

Journal your thoughts

Day 30

Then he said to me, "Prophesy to the breath; prophesy, son of man, and say to the breath, Thus says the Lord God: Come from the four winds, O breath, and breathe on these slain, that they may live." Ezekiel 37:9 ESV

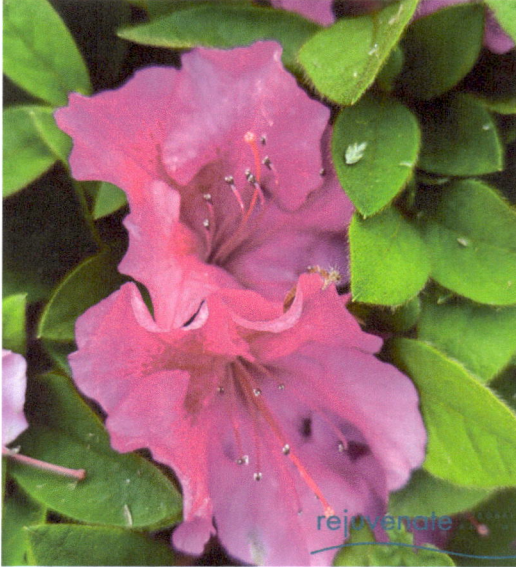

Today's Intentions:

1. Express gratitude for the journey and the lessons learned along the way.
2. Reflect on personal growth and celebrate the milestones achieved.
3. Set intentions for the future, embodying a sense of purpose and direction.

Reflections:

- Expressing gratitude for the journey fills you with a profound sense of appreciation for the experiences, challenges, and blessings that have shaped you into who you are today.

- Reflecting on personal growth allows you to celebrate the progress made and acknowledge the inner strength and resilience that have carried you through both triumphs and tribulations.

- Setting intentions for the future fills you with excitement and determination, guiding you towards a life filled with purpose, passion, and fulfillment.

Journal your thoughts

Journal your thoughts

Journal your thoughts

Journal your thoughts

Journal your thoughts

Journal your thoughts

_____

_____

_____

_____

_____

_____

_____

_____

_____

_____

_____

_____

_____

_____

_____

Biography

Dr. Chichi Nwankwo Ezeike is a multifaceted professional and a beacon of inspiration in the fields of health and wellness. Born in Houston, TX, and raised in Nigeria, Dr. Chichi's journey is marked by resilience, dedication, and a passion for holistic health.

A personal battle with hypertension led Dr. Chichi to explore holistic health solutions, culminating in her certification as a Health Coach. Combining her medical knowledge with health coaching principles, she founded Rejuvenate Integrative Health and Wellness. Her practice offers personalized wellness plans tailored to individual needs, helping clients manage hypertension, diabetes, weight loss, and nutritional goals. Dr. Chichi's approach emphasizes bio-individuality, recognizing that each person's path to health is unique.

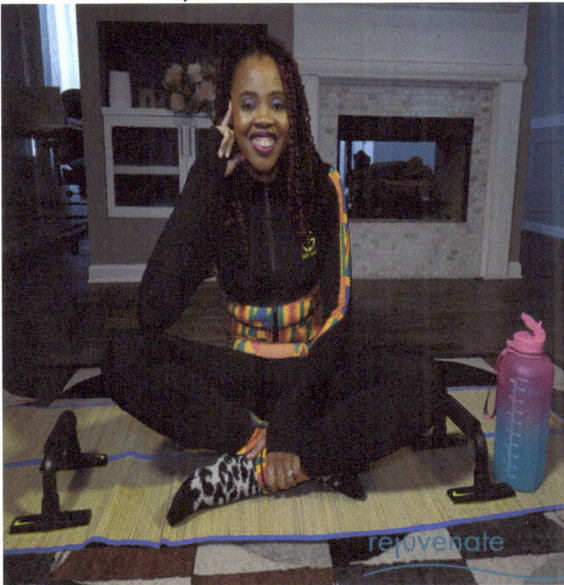

At Rejuvenate Integrative Health and Wellness, Dr. Chichi guides clients through various wellness aspects, including healthy recipes, mindfulness practices, and reflective journaling. She advocates for a balanced lifestyle, encouraging clients to listen to their bodies, honor their needs, and celebrate small victories on their health journeys.

In her personal life, Dr. Chichi enjoys working out, nature walks, family time, traveling, cooking, and swimming. Her multifaceted roles as a health coach, educator, entrepreneur, and community advocate makes her a dynamic force dedicated to improving lives through holistic wellness.

Other books co-authored by Dr. Chichi:

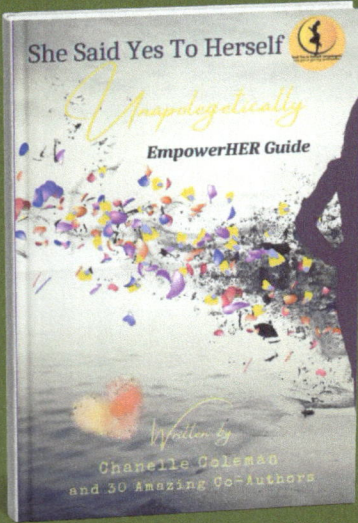

She Said Yes To Herself Unapologetically

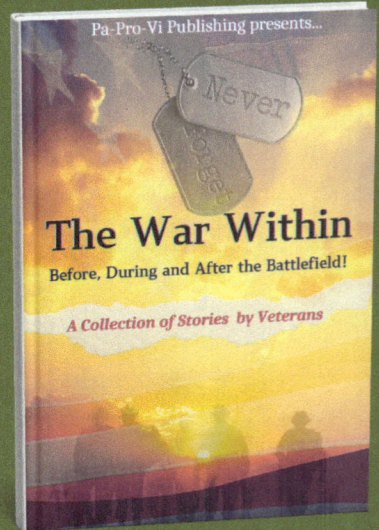

The War Within, Before, During and After the Battlefield

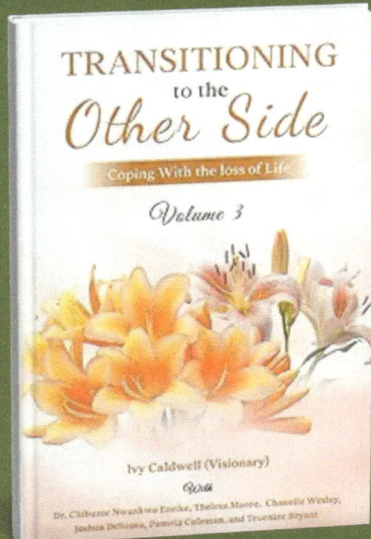

Transitioning to the Other Side Volume 3

www.ingramcontent.com/pod-product-compliance
Lightning Source LLC
Chambersburg PA
CBHW041217270326
41931CB00001B/16